I0483004

The Art of Self-Adjusting

Michael Hetherington
(L. Ac, Yoga Teacher)

Copyright 2013 Michael Hetherington

By law this work is protected by copyright and therefore no one is permitted to copy, broadcast, transmit, show or play in public, adapt or change in any way the content of this e-book for any other purpose whatsoever without the prior written permission from Michael Hetherington.

www.michaelhetherington.com.au

info@michaelhetherington.com.au

Australia

Disclaimer

All material in this book is provided for your information only and may not be construed as medical advice or instruction. No action or inaction should be taken based solely on the contents of this information; instead, readers should consult appropriate health professionals on any matter relating to their health and well-being.

The information and opinions expressed here are believed to be accurate, based on the best judgment available to the authors, and readers who fail to consult with appropriate health authorities assume the risk of any injuries. The publisher is not responsible for errors or omissions.

*"Every human being is the author of his
own health or disease."*

~ Buddha

About the Author

Michael Hetherington is a qualified acupuncturist, health practitioner and yoga teacher based in Brisbane, Australia. He has a keen interest in mind-body medicine, energetic anatomy, nutrition and herbs, yoga nidra, and Buddhist-style meditation. Inspired by the teachings of many, he has learned that a light-hearted, joyful approach to life serves best.

Other Titles by Author:

Chakra Balancing Made Simple and Easy

Meditation Made Simple

How to Do Restorative Yoga

Autumn Oriental Yoga

The Little Book of Yin

How to Learn Acupuncture

Table of Contents

Introduction

While self-adjustment is no substitute for the expert knowledge and experience of a health professional, a great deal of benefit and enhanced musculoskeletal health can be acquired by simply practicing a set of simple self-healthcare techniques and practices. The benefits of being able to manage your own musculoskeletal health include but are not limited to:

- Less pain
- The reduction of reliance on pain-reducing medications
- More physical and mental energy
- A deeper connection with your body
- Easier and more efficient movement
- The saving of money due to the reduction in health-related appointments
- Better overall health and well-being

The purpose of this book is to explain some basic fundamental principles in relation to managing your body, spine, and posture for greater health. It also goes into various techniques one can do to release tightness and compression throughout the body. Throughout this book, I have primarily focused on the health of the lumbar spine (lower back) and thoracic spine (upper back). Due to the complexity and fragility of the cervical spine, I have chosen to leave it out. The neck is a very fragile area of the spine, therefore it is recommended that you seek help from a qualified osteopath or chiropractor to have any neck adjustments performed.

In this book you will learn:

- A simple five-step process for self-adjusting.
- More about one of the most important and undervalued tissues in the musculoskeletal system— the connective tissue.
- Three yoga-style stretches that anyone can do right now to help decompress the spine and prepare for a self–adjustment.
- Tools and tips that help to release muscles and connective tissues.
- Supplements for a healthier musculoskeletal system.
- How to begin retraining your musculoskeletal system for more efficient movements that provide long-term solutions to many pain problems.

The five steps that will be discussed in detail throughout this book are:

1. *Relax and release the musculature*

2. *Soften and lengthen connective tissue*

3. *Twist to adjust (with or without a "pop")*

4. *Lubricate and nourish*

5. *Reorganize the body for more efficient movement*

Spinal Anatomy 101

The spinal system is comprised of bones, nerves, cartilage, muscles, and large amounts of connective tissue. The purpose of the boney structure of the spine is to protect the spinal cord that runs throughout the spinal column. It also provides attachment points for the muscles and connective tissues. The movement of the spine is largely controlled by the contraction of muscles that are attached to the spine.

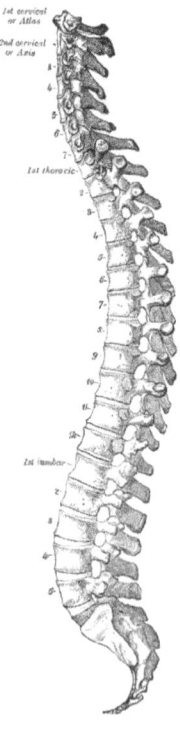

The spine is comprised of thirty-three individual bones called vertebrae, of which, five are fused together in the sacrum area of the spinal column. They are grouped into four regions: The cervical spine, which is comprised of seven vertebrae, is located at the top of the spinal column, and directly supports the skull; The thoracic spine, which is comprised of twelve vertebrae, has the twelve ribs attached, and is located in the upper-back region of the body; The lumbar spine, which is comprised of five vertebrae, and is located in the lower back; and the sacrum, which is comprised of five vertebrae which are fused into a triangular shape at the base of the spine, and is attached to the pelvic region. The coccyx, which is comprised of three very small vertebrae, attaches to the bottom of the sacrum.

In between each of the vertebrae exist discs of fibrous cartilage and connective tissues that act as cushioning and shock-absorbing pads. These pads are called "intervertebral fibrocartilage".

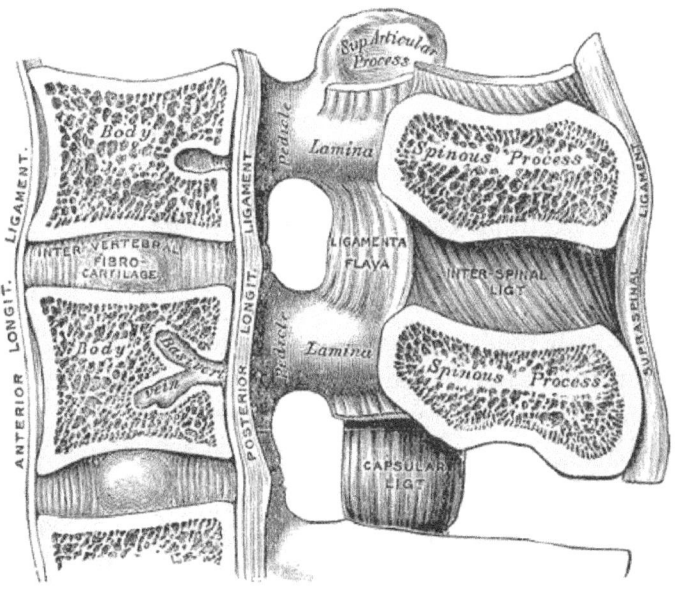

Spinal nerves travel through the center of the spinal column and branch out from there to access the organs and other tissues of the body so that the nervous system and brain can communicate effectively. Any injury or impairment of these nerves can lead to all sorts of health problems and pain-related symptoms. Therefore, keeping your spinal column and nerves in good condition is paramount if you wish to live a healthy and pain-free life.

The Slipped Disc Explained

Before we go any further, it is important to clarify what a slipped disc is. A slipped disc does not mean that a vertebra has "slipped" out of its position. What it means is that the intervertebral fibrocartilage disc that is located between the vertebral discs has become stressed, overly compressed, or weakened, and is protruding out in some direction. This often results in pressure upon one of the nerve branches coming out of the spinal column. It can be caused by a number factors, from a lack of water and fluid in the connective tissues to bending awkwardly, heavy lifting, too much sitting, poor posture, inefficient movement behavior, the lack of movement and stretching of muscles and tissues around the spine, being overweight, weight-bearing sports, and traumatic-type injuries or accidents. The most common area for slipped discs is in the lumbar region of the spine, around L3 – L5.

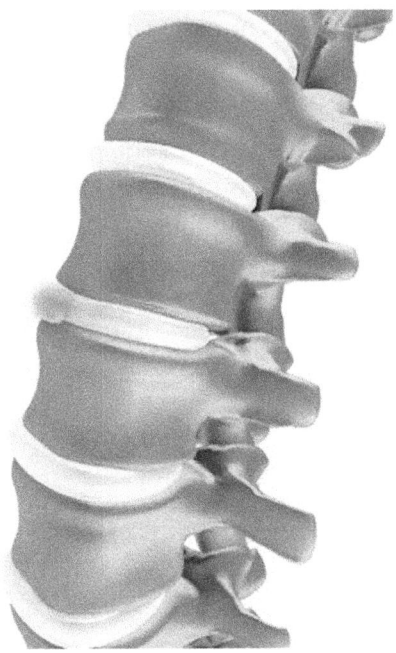

A photo on a spine model showing an intervertebral disc protruding out the side and potentially pinching a nerve.

Often, if compression is the sole cause of a slipped disc, all that is required for the disc to return to its proper position is to decompress the vertebral bones. This is done by relaxing the muscles and lengthening the connective tissues in the area. About 99% of the time, the disc will return to its natural position if given the space to do so. You can be proactive in this approach by taking the time to practice deep stretching to relax the muscles and stretch the connective tissue, engaging in gentle movements to help move blood and nutrients into the area, taking adequate fluids and nutrition to nourish the body, and getting enough rest. It is best to avoid adding any extra stress, tension, or dehydration, and to avoid sitting in poorly-designed furniture for extended periods.

If you are suffering from a slipped disc, be sure to explore a variety of options for treatment and rehabilitation. I would encourage you to utilize the best of both eastern and western medicine alongside one another for the best and quickest results. In regards to the techniques outlined in this book, I would only advise the practice of deep stretching (yin yoga) to lengthen connective tissue, and the use of supplementation.

Hyper-Mobile Joints and Cracking

The popping sound produced when you crack your knuckles or get an adjustment by a chiropractor has baffled medical scientists for many decades. These days, however, the most common understanding and theory to explain the popping sound is that it is produced from something called cavitation. This means that there are fluids inside of a space, and then a sudden change of pressure occurs. In other words, it is where the pressure of the liquid falls below its vapor pressure. This is similar to what happens when you open a can of soda, or when you lift a glass of water off a table where fluid has formed around its base, causing a kind of suction cup and producing a slight popping sound as you lift it up off the table.

Many people have a regular type of stretch or movement that produces a crack or a pop within their body somewhere. Often, it can provide us with some relief, and therefore the tendency is to do it regularly and to do it often. This is not always the best approach or practice to do continuously because when we regularly crack the same joint, what is usually happening is that that particular joint becomes hyper-mobile, meaning over-flexible. Being hyper-mobile or over-flexible is not such a great thing, because it can easily allow the ligaments and tissues around the joints to overstretch, which can lead to joint pain, joint inflammation, and tendinitis, and dramatically increases the chance of injury down the track.

A small number of people are hyper-mobile all throughout their bodies, and seem to be extremely flexible. This is when a person will be able to do many yoga-style stretches with ease, or look like a gymnast—but if they are not activating their muscles correctly to protect their joints, all the stretching will actually cause them joint problems in the future. Therefore, the advanced-looking yoga poses are not necessarily a healthy or suitable practice. In most cases they will need to work at pulling back their practice, and re-learning the basics of proper alignment and muscular activation to avoid overextending their joints.

Most of us, however, are not hyper-flexible in the body—but we are likely to be hyper-mobile in just a few joints of the body. These are the joints that we regularly crack or pop to get some relief every now and then. Because this practice leads to hyper-mobile joints, it is not the best practice to continue. In most cases there is a joint (or a series of joints) around the hyper-mobile joint that needs the attention, but because the hyper-mobile joint is moving so freely, it takes all the attention and mobility away from the stiff, immobile joints. This is why a professional may need to be called in every now and then to get some movement back into the hard-to-get areas and joints. It is possible to get into these hard-to-get places ourselves if we take the time out to soften the tissues of the body, and if we follow the techniques and steps outlined in the following chapters.

"Blessed are the flexible, for they shall not be bent out of shape."

~ Unknown

The Fundamentals of Self-Adjustment

The five steps to self-adjusting are:

1. Soften and relax the musculature

2. Soften and lengthen connective tissue

3. Twist to adjust (with or without a "pop")

4. Lubricate and nourish

5. Reorganize body for more efficient movement

1. Soften and Relax the Musculature

Because bones are held in place by muscles and connective tissues, it is a fundamental principle that these tissues need to be softened and relaxed before any adjustment takes place. Muscles generally react more quickly than connective tissue, and most muscles can be released from their tension state after a good few breaths and the application of the right pressure in the right spot. The most reactive spots tend to be "trigger points" or "acupressure points". You know you've found a trigger point when there is an intense, uncomfortable muscular sensation, followed by some kind of tingling sensation, experienced either around the same area or in another area of the body not apparently related.

Applying pressure to these muscles sends a signal to the brain, which then sends a signal back to the muscle to release and lengthen. If the tightness in the muscle has only been accumulated within a day or two of adjustment, the muscle will quickly unlock and release itself without much effort.

Muscles that have been contracted for long periods of time (over two weeks) will tend to stiffen up and crystallize into hardened areas of tissue. This impairs the flow of blood and nutrients into that area. This lack of blood flow and nutrients to the area greatly affects the capacity for the body to heal and repair itself. These areas will release a little, but tend to remain as hardened tissue even after the associated trigger point has been activated and worked on. These locked-up tissues become a source of stagnated potential energy. It can take a long time for the crystallized structures to break down, and for blood and nutrients to flush the area for proper repair. It will require a variety of approaches that may include applying heat (hot shower, burning moxa, heat packs), massage, stretching, exercise, acupuncture, and proper diet to give these muscles the best opportunity to release from this state and reduce overall stiffness.

If the muscles aren't softened and relaxed, it is very likely that an adjustment won't "hold" for very long. This often results in the bone or its associated tissues returning to the position it was in prior to the adjustment. Therefore, muscle tissue NEEDS to be released and relaxed before an effective adjustment can take place.

Because we are mainly focusing on the back, applying massage will require a second person. While this is recommended, it is a luxury that is not always available or affordable. Finding a good massage therapist is not always easy either, and it is not recommended to just go to anyone you find in the local newspaper. Because this book is focused on self-adjustment, we will explore ways to relax the musculature without the need for a second person.

On the next page is a picture of the most common trigger or acupressure points on the back.

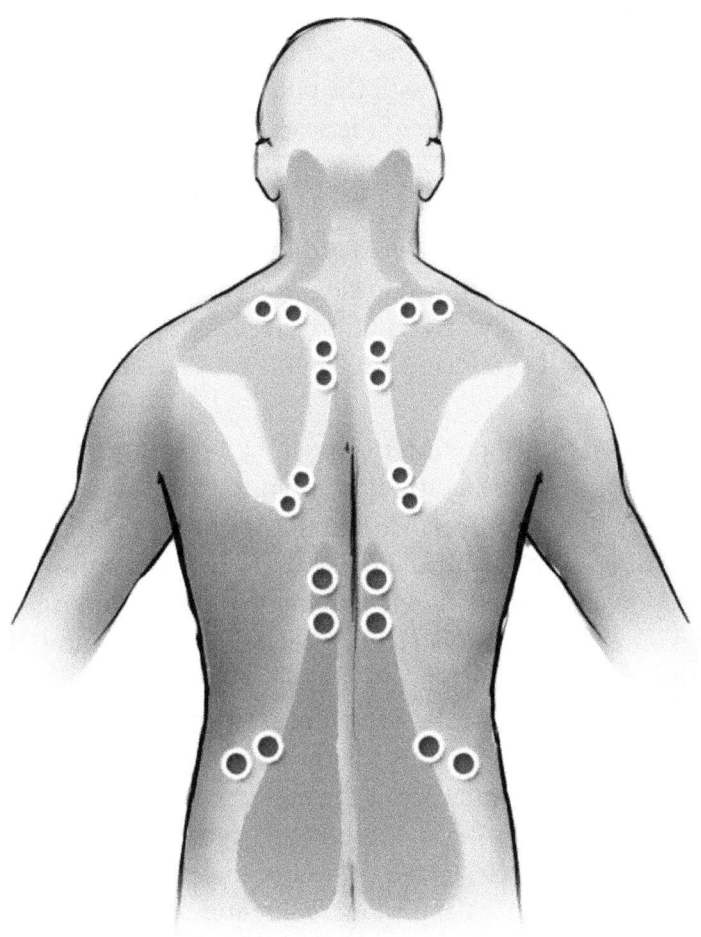

One method to access these trigger points is to lay on a tennis ball and move your weight around until you find "the spots". If a tennis ball doesn't work for you, you can try things like "bak balls" (www.bakballs.com), or better still, start experimenting with items around the house.

I have also found that long-poled items like broom handles or pieces of bamboo can be used by holding the pole behind your back with your hands at either end, and applying pressure to various points on the back with the pole. It works especially well for the points across the top of the scapula and shoulders.

Another idea is to simply use the external corner of a wall to lean your back up against. This works great for the points in between the shoulder blades. Simply adjust your weight and lean back into the corner of the wall when you find a reactive point. When found, take long deep breaths to help the muscle release.

Whenever you locate a point, the most important thing to do is to get in touch with your breathing. Use your exhale breath the most, and imagine that you are literally breathing the tightness out of your body. Naturally, because of the intense sensation produced, your awareness of the area of your body that is being worked on will increase—so let it. Keep focusing on your breath, and the area of the body being worked on. Continue to let the area go; let it sink; let it relax as you breathe out. If you are doing it correctly, it will usually only take about 5 – 10 breaths to completely clear the intensity of the area and release the muscle. But again, if it's a long-term condition of tightness in a particular muscle or set of muscles, it won't release completely no matter how much pressure you apply and will require a more multi-leveled approach, as previously mentioned.

Stretching can also quickly release tight muscle fibers. Again, because muscle fibers tend to react quickly, you can come into a stretch and then use your breath and awareness of the area to release and relax the muscle. Forward bends work especially well for opening up the back of the body and the shoulder blades.

2. Gently Lengthen Connective Tissue to Decompress Joints and Bones

This second step is focused more on the connective tissue of the body. Unlike the muscles of the body that tend to respond quickly, connective tissue takes time to soften and relax. The best and most effective way to access the connective tissues is through long and sustained stretching, which involves holding a stretch in a relaxed yet supported state for at least 3 – 5 minutes. This is the type of stretching and approach to exercise that 99% of people don't do.

Around every joint (knee, elbow, wrist, ankle, etc.) and vertebral disc are layers and layers of connective tissues. Connective tissue is like a plastic wrap that surrounds all the organs and bones in the body, therefore making it one of the most important tissues in the body. Previously, connective tissue has been looked over by medical scientists as simply a tissue that holds things in place. More recently, though, it has been discovered that connective tissue is involved in a vast number of functions, and has a very important role in keeping all the tissues in the body in a healthy state.

The causes of many conditions like chronic fatigue, fibromyalgia, chronic lower back pain, ongoing headaches and other musculoskeletal related conditions I believe are also strongly associated with connective tissue stress and tightness, and therefore can be more effectively treated if we learn to lengthen and nourish the connective tissues more effectively within the body.

Due to the natural tendency for compression to occur in the lower back, especially from sitting for long hours, the connective tissue tends to shorten into a new, shortened length. Over time, this connective tissue tightness and shrunken length will likely contribute to a slipped disc, or associated symptoms that involve the ongoing compression of the vertebral discs. Therefore, the most effective, natural, and healthy way to free yourself from this compression is to stretch the connective tissue in the area. We are essentially aiming to create more space between the joints. The most practical way to do this would be a method called "yin yoga", while other things like inversion tables and other contraptions can also be of help.

The basic principle with connective tissue stretching is that you need to completely relax the musculature in the area so that the connective tissue can be accessed and lengthened. The following descriptions and postures will help guide you into stretches that aim to lengthen the connective tissue specifically. Remember, you need to hold the poses for at least three minutes each to allow the connective tissues to respond.

With the following stretches, we are only aiming to generate moderate stress on the tissues by stretching and lengthening them. The aim is not to "push through" the pain and go to your maximum. If your breath becomes really short or strained, or if you experience any sharp shooting sensations, you are going too hard—so back off! Use your breath to guide you. After some time in the stretch, the sensations will probably change location in the body as different tissues are being accessed. This is a good sign; it means that it is getting deeper, and into new areas of the body.

The other important thing about this type of stretching is that it generally is not a comfortable feeling sitting with an intense sensation for three minutes. It's easy for the mind to talk you into pulling out after just a minute or two, telling you, "you've done enough", "this is boring", or "this is too much, I can't do it". It is important to stay in the stretch even when the mind is having a go at you, because this type of stretching is a type of mental training also. Learning to deal with and be okay with uncomfortable sensations is a valuable skill to have in life. Life is not always comfortable or easy, and by using these types of stretches we can train ourselves to be okay with a little bit of discomfort or uneasiness without reacting strongly to it in mind. Remember this next time you are holding your next deep stretch.

If you experience any sharp shooting sensations while practicing the following stretches then back off and stop immediately. I this happens to you then it is advisable to seek help from health professional such as an osteopath.

Connective Tissue Stretches

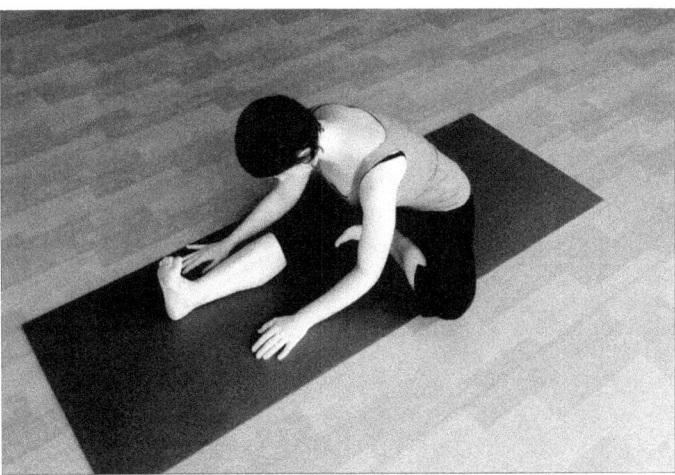

One-legged forward bend

1. Begin by sitting on the floor or mat. If you find your lower back curls behind you, or if you have difficultly sitting on the floor, then sit up on some folded blankets or a small pillow. This slight

elevation helps align the hips and takes the strain out of the lower back.

2. Bend the right knee and place the right foot on the inside of the left leg. If your right knee hurts for any reason, you can place a pillow or folded blanket under the right knee. Be sure to look after your knee joint!

3. Then, simply inhale and lengthen your spine. As you exhale, bring your chest and heart space forward and down toward the left leg.

4. You are going to be in this position for some time, so take your time getting into it. Allow your breath to guide you. Relax your shoulders and eventually bring the head down, even tucking the chin slightly into the chest. Relax your body, legs, arms, head, and neck. Let gravity do the work for you. Just keep focused on letting it go so that the tissues can lengthen.

5. Hold for at least three minutes. When you're ready to come out, slowly ease yourself up using your hands for support.

6. Once you are out of the pose, feel free to have a gentle wiggle by bending the knees up and drawing them gently from side to side to release any feelings of stagnation.

7. When ready, repeat on the other side.

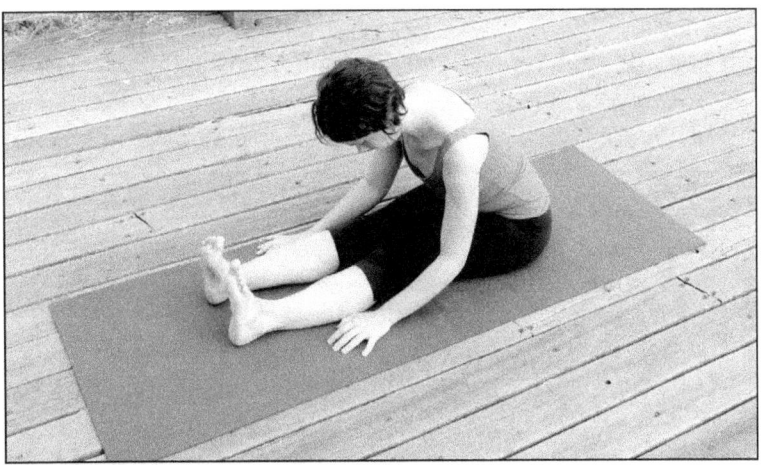

Seated forward bend

1. Be sure to have completed the previous pose so that this stretch will come easier to your body.

2. To start, sit on the floor or mat. Again, if your lower back rounds out or it feels really awkward and uncomfortable, sit up on some folded blankets or a form pillow.

3. Bring both legs out in front.

4. Inhale to lengthen your torso and spine, then as you exhale, start to draw your chest and heart space forward and down towards the legs.

5. Take your time getting into it. Eventually, relax your shoulders, put your head down, relax your legs, and let gravity take over. It helps to close the eyes to go deeply into it.

6. Hold for at least three minutes.

7. When you are ready to come up, draw yourself up slowly, using your hands for extra support.

8. When you are up, have a wiggle to remove any stagnation.

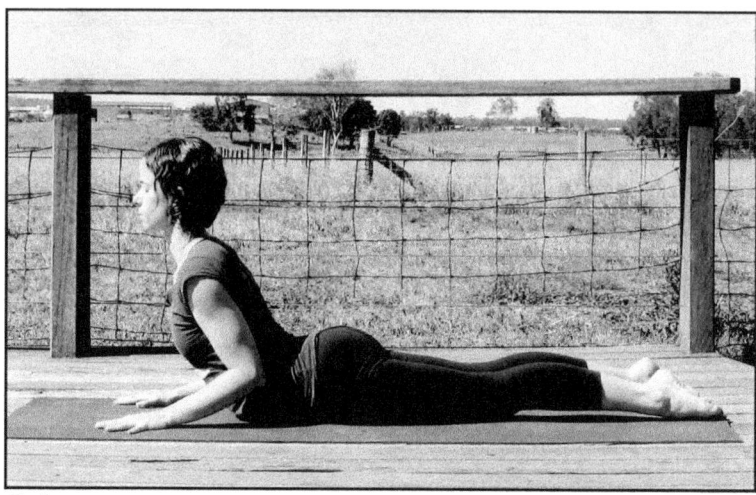

Cobra

1.To help bend the spine in the other direction, we do the cobra after a series of forward bends. It feels amazing after the forward bends!

2. To begin, lay on your belly. Relax your head, and just have a little moment to settle on the mat.

3. When you are ready, draw your elbows under your shoulders and have your palms out in front of you, facing down. If the palms don't face down easily, then up is okay too.

4. Get the sense of lifting your chest so that it can open; be sure not to simply sink into the shoulders.

5. Once you are there, focus on relaxing your buttocks, legs, and lower back completely. Let gravity sink into your lower back.

6. The only real activation is through the shoulders to hold you up. You can experiment a little with the head placement, either looking forward and up (be sure to lengthen the back of the neck by giving yourself a double chin, as this keeps the muscles in the neck long and avoids the compression that can occur in the back of the head), or by bringing the head down, with the chin towards chest if that feels better.

7. You usually don't need to stay in this pose for as long as the others, and three minutes is often more than enough. Anywhere from 1 – 3 minutes is recommended.

8. When you are ready to come out, simply release your elbows and rest yourself down on your belly. Allow the lower back to settle.

9. Have a wiggle of the hips to remove any stagnation.

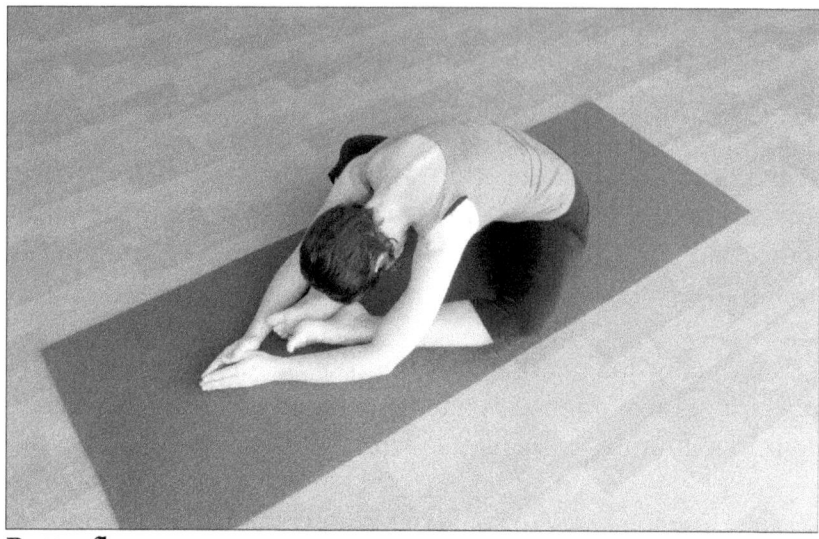

Butterfly

1. Come down onto the mat or floor and bring the soles of the feet together. Allow a comfortable space between your groin and your feet so that your legs come to make a diamond shape.

2. Try to lengthen through your lower back as you grab hold of your feet, before you start to come forward over the legs.

3. Draw your torso, your belly, your chest and eventually your head down towards the floor. Take your time, don't rush! Eventually move your arms and hands into a comfortable position so that you can stay in this posture for at least 3 minutes.

4. Find your breath through the nose, relax your shoulders, arms and legs. Allow yourself to sink into the pose.

5. After at least 3 minutes slowly guide yourself back up to a seated position and relax your posture.

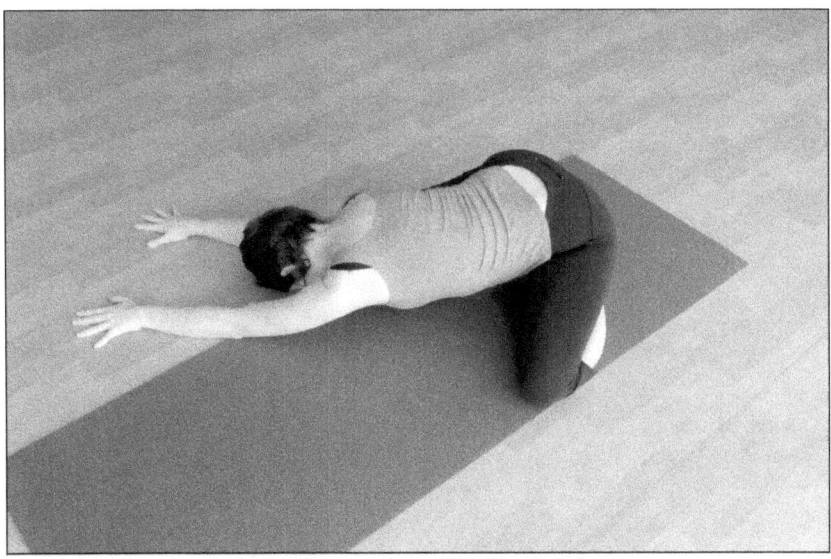

Knees Wide with Side Extension (Right Side)

1. Come to sit on your heels, tops of the fleet flat. If this creates any sharp shooting painful sensations in your ankles or knees, back off and try placing a blanket under the feet or between your heels and buttocks. Please note, if this pose is still painful even after adding a blanket, than avoid this posture altogether.

2. Bring the knees wide. Start to draw your torso forwards and down, bring the arms out in front and walk your arms over to the right side so that your torso is heading towards your right thigh.

3. Continue to draw yourself forward and down, extending the arms out towards the right side. Extend the left arm so that you feel a stretch up through the side of your torso. Relax your head and neck downwards. Hold for a few minutes, softening your body with each exhale.

3. After a few minutes slowly draw yourself up using your hands for support. Relax and release your posture if you need to.

4. Repeat the stretch to the other side.

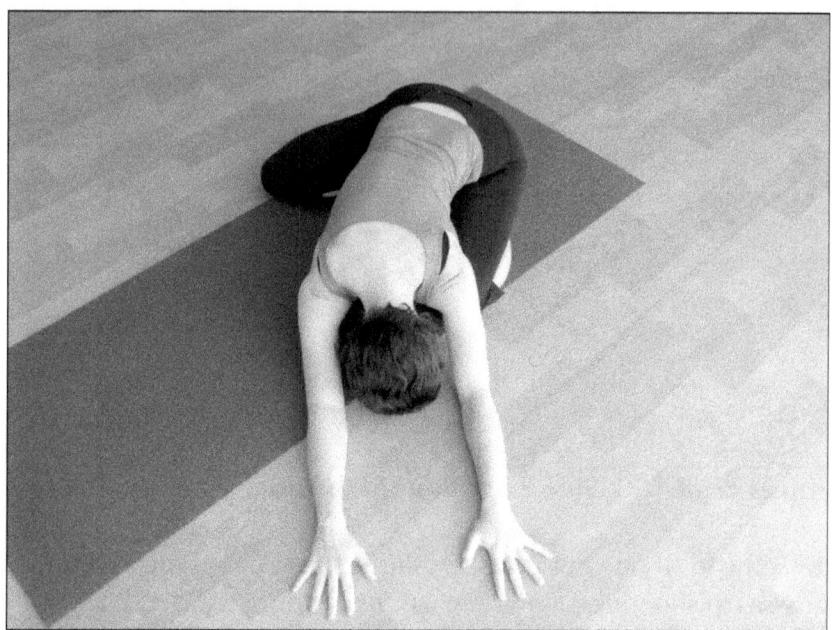

Knees Wide with Side Extension (Left Side)

4. Repeat the instructions from the previous stretch, this time however, move the torso towards the left side.

3. After a few minutes slowly draw yourself up using your hands for support. Relax and release your posture if you need to.

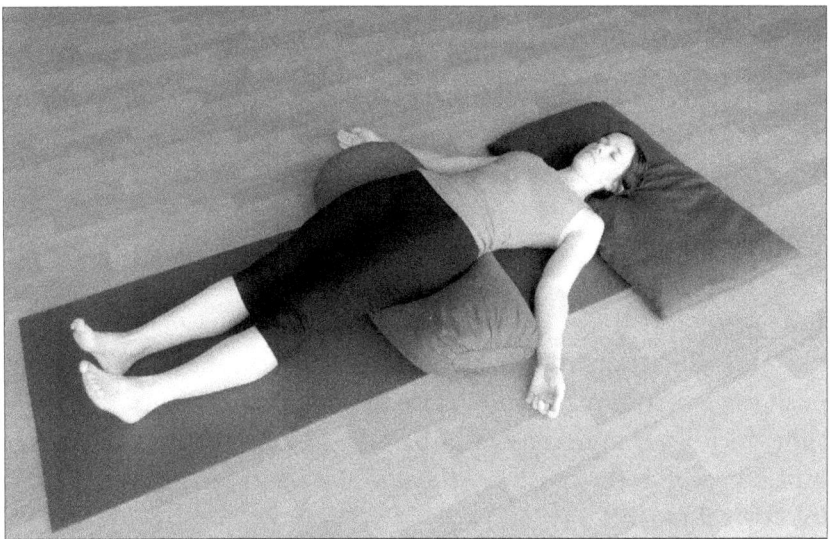

Supported Hips Pose

1. Sit up naturally on your mat and bring the bolster crosswise into the middle of your mat.

2. Sit on top of the bolster with your knees bent.

3. When you're ready, slowly lower your back and torso towards the floor, using your arms for support. (There is another way to get into this position, which I have explained in the "variations" section that comes next.)

4. Make sure your shoulders rest comfortably on the floor. Also, make sure that the bolster is comfortably in your lower back curve; don't let it come up to touch the lower ribs.

5. Make sure your sacrum and your hips sit comfortably on the bolster.

6. You can bring a folded blanket under the back of your head if you wish.

7. You can keep your knees bent, or, some people like to extend the legs out straight. Do whatever feels good for you.

8. Stay here as long as comfortable, at least 2 – 3 minutes.

Variation:

1. Another way to get into this pose that may be easier for you is to simply lie flat on your back on the floor. Then bend the knees, push the feet into the floor to raise the hips towards the sky, and slide the bolster in underneath the sacrum and hip area. Relax the hips down onto the bolster. Adjust as necessary; check step four for correct positioning.

The Best Tool—The Gym Ball

I have found that the gym ball is the best tool for lengthening connective tissue. Remember though, to be effective at lengthening the connective tissue, you need to hold the pose for at least three minutes. It can become intense after a minute or so if the connective tissue is releasing. It can feel like the bones are being gently pulled apart, or like there is a vacuum of intense energy being unlocked in the middle of it all. You have to realize that some connective tissues have not been stretched in that way for a long time—maybe even your entire lifetime. Just keep your breath moving, and keep focusing on relaxing and letting the sensation run its course.

What often happens during these stretches is that after a few minutes, the sensation tends to "run out", or dissipate greatly from its original intensity. In many cases, especially if the area being stretched and worked on is a "weak spot" or an area that we compress easily due to our movement behavior, it will continue to produce intense sensations when doing this type of stretching over many weeks, months, or even years. Sometimes it will heal completely, and the intense sensations will completely dissipate— and sometimes it won't leave us completely. Regardless of the full outcome, it will help to reduce any pain, and it will support the process of healing in that area of the body. Therefore, it should be considered a practice of body maintenance as well as self-rehabilitation.

Here is a list of stretches you can easily do on a gym ball at home. Make sure the gym ball isn't too big for you; you want to be able to easily stabilize yourself with your legs on the floor.

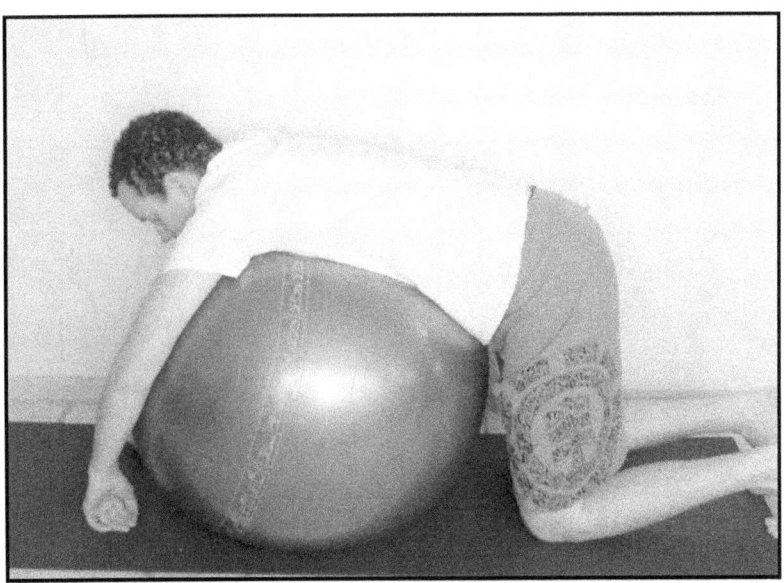

To Stretch the Upper Back and Between the Shoulder Blades

1. Simply bring the ball under the chest area. You can make slight adjustments to the ball to find a position where you start to feel a release occurring in the upper back.

2. Once a comfortable and releasing position is found, focus on relaxing your shoulders, arms, head, and lower body. Let gravity take over. Closing the eyes helps a lot in letting go.

3. Hold for at least three minutes.

4. When you are ready to come up, slowly roll back towards the knees, and gently draw yourself up using your hands.

5. If you feel unsteady or dizzy in any way, take a seat, have a sip of water, and take your time to regain your senses.

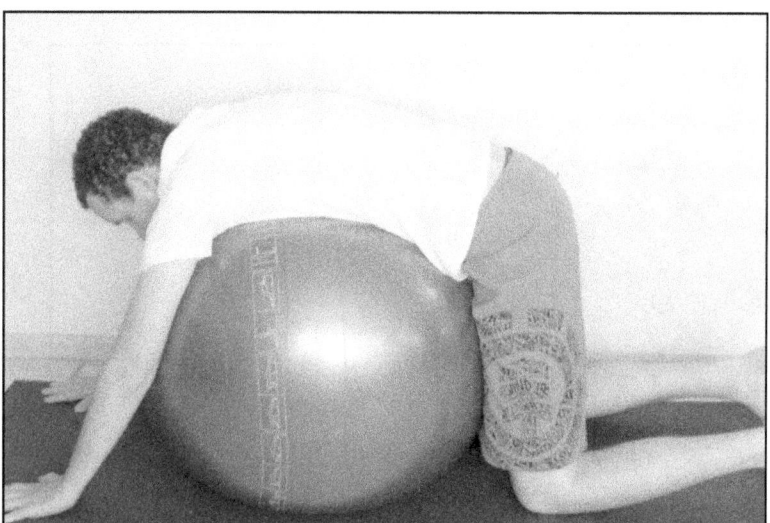

To Stretch the Middle Back

1. Bring the ball into the middle of your torso. You can make slight adjustments of the ball to find a position where you start to feel a release occurring in the middle of the back.

2. Once a comfortable and releasing position is found, focus on relaxing your shoulders, arms, head, and lower body. Let gravity take over. Closing the eyes helps a lot in letting go.

3. Hold for at least three minutes.

4. When you are ready to come up, slowly roll back towards the knees, and gently draw yourself up using your hands.

5. If you feel unsteady or dizzy in any way, take a seat, have a sip of water, and take your time to regain your senses.

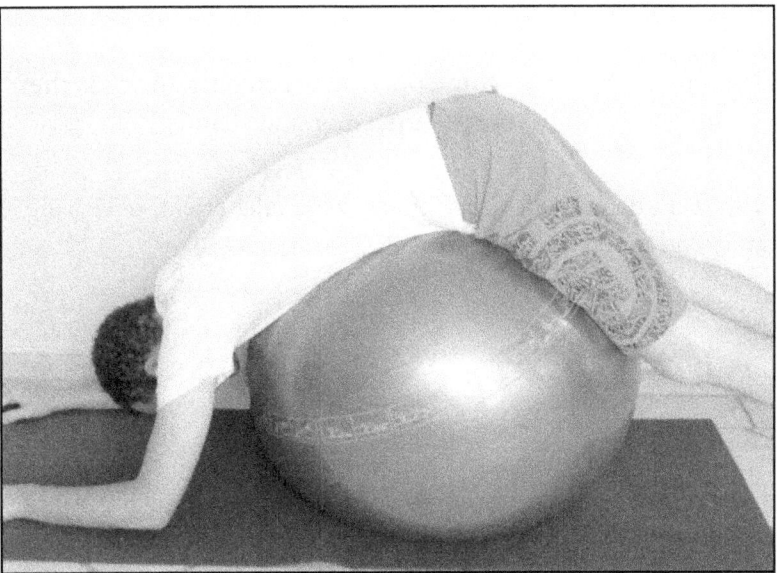

To Stretch and Open the Lower Back

This one is a little more dynamic, as it requires a bit more effort in balancing with the arms, and it also involves an inversion, meaning the head will be lower than the heart and will produce a blood rush to the head. Therefore, if you have high blood pressure, feel free to come out when you feel like you've had enough rather than waiting for the full three minutes to pass.

1. Bring the ball into the lower belly area. You can make slight adjustments to the ball to find a position where you start to feel a release occurring in the lower back and sacrum area.

2. Once a comfortable and releasing position is found, focus on relaxing your shoulders, arms, head, and lower body. Let gravity take over. Closing the eyes helps a lot in letting go.

3. Hold for at least three minutes.

4. When you are ready to come up, slowly roll back towards the knees, and gently draw yourself up using your hands.

5. If you feel unsteady or dizzy in any way, take a seat, have a sip of water, and take your time to regain your senses.

The Full (and Intense) Inversion Practice

There are other ways to access connective tissue besides doing yoga-style stretches. The most obvious method is by using some kind of inversion apparatus. There are many on the market, and they have been around since the 1970s. I prefer to use a yoga swing. Be sure to get some instruction from a qualified trainer before attempting full inversions, as there is often a few tips and tricks they will provide you to make the experience much smoother.

I attended many classes in aerial yoga before I bought a yoga swing and attempted it at home. There is no doubt that full inversions are intense experiences. In aerial yoga, they recommend being in the full inversion for about ten minutes to gain the full benefits. This gives the body enough time to regulate the blood flow and flush all the tissues with fluids. I always recommend doing a warm-up of at least ten minutes of exercise or stretching before going into any full inversion. That way, the muscles are warm and the blood is flowing; this will reduce the shock of the inversion to the body.

Caution: Inversion is not recommended for those who are pregnant, or who have high blood pressure, heart conditions, or eye problems.

Some people who are new to the practice may experience a headache after doing a full inversion due to the detoxifying effect that the flushing of the body fluids creates.

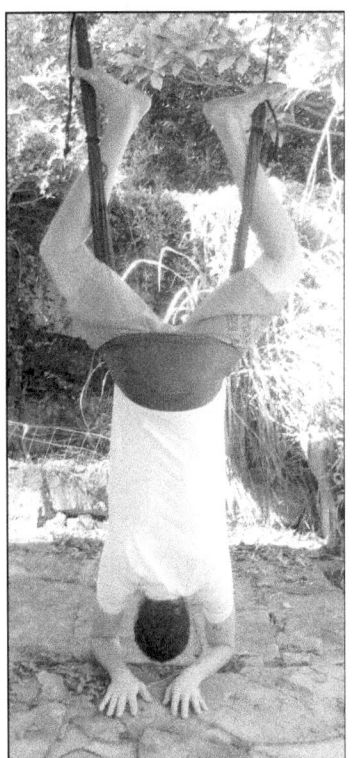

Yoga Swing Inversion

1. Only attempt a full inversion after you have done a ten-minute warm-up, and have received proper, real-life instruction from a professional trainer on how to get into a full inversion.

2. When you are in the inversion, try placing the backs of the hands on the floor, as this tends to reduce any feelings of anxiety or panic that may come up.

3. Then, focus on relaxing the lower back, shoulders, legs, and entire body.

4. Keep your breath steady and smooth. Allow the body to do its thing.

5. When you feel ready to come up, slowly draw yourself up using the method explained by your trainer.

6. Be sure to rest; allow the head to rest downwards so the blood flow to the body can be restored before attempting to walk or do anything else.

7. Have a sip of water, and take your time to get back your senses.

Spinal Decompression Tables

These are modified tables that you basically get strapped onto, and then parts of your spine are gently, systematically, and continuously pulled apart by a controlled, mechanical device. This type of treatment has been around since the 1980s, and has been recommended to many as a non-surgical option for those with serious spinal compression. With what little research has been conducted on this type of treatment, it is reported to have a 70 – 80% success rate in reducing back pain caused from compression. One of the main obstacles to this form of treatment is the price tag, as it will cost anywhere from $2000 – $5000 for a series of twenty treatments.

The principle of slowly and continuously lengthening the connective tissue to pry apart the compressed bones is exactly the same principle used in yin yoga and inversion therapy, and therefore I would recommend trying out these other methods before considering using spinal decompression tables.

3. Twist to Adjust

Once the musculature is relaxed and the connective tissue is lengthened creating more space between the joints, it will be much easier to get an adjustment. Also, it is best if the body is in a slightly warm state, either after a series of stretching, some gentle exercise or after having a hot shower or bath as this allows the tissues to be more elastic and it also allows the blood and fluids to flow throughout the body much easier.

When you go for the adjustment, you may get a popping or cracking sound, and you may not. It's not the goal here to get a sound. Sometimes things can move into new positions without a crack or a pop, so don't push it or aim for a sound to occur every time.

The adjustment of any bone or tissue in this method largely depends on the notion of "the body's own intelligence". This means that if you can create enough space for a movement to occur, the body will move whatever it is into its rightful place on its own, due to its own "intelligence". Therefore, our focus is just to get things to relax and support the movement process using these techniques; the body takes care of the rest for us.

To make an adjustment, come into one of the supported twist poses outlined below. When moving into the pose, be sure to go in slowly, and allow the movement to twist from your lower back and slowly move up to the neck area. Get a sense that you are able to slightly move each individual vertebra from the base up as you twist. *When moving into any twist, be sure to move into the twist on the exhale, not the inhale.*

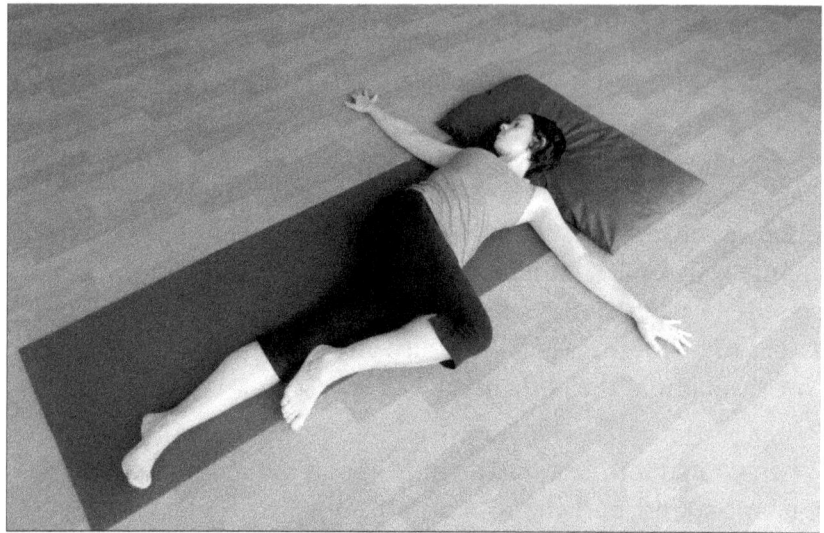

The Simple Twist

1. To begin, lie on the floor or mat with both legs extended.

2. Then, bend your left knee, and place your left foot gently on top of your right knee.

3. Place your left arm out to the side at about shoulder height, and your right hand on top of your left knee.

4. Now draw the left knee across your body using your right hand for support. You may get a pop or you may not; both are ok. This movement is effectively adjusting the bone while twisting and squeezing the muscles and connective tissues in the back of the body.

5. If your neck is okay, look towards your left arm.

6. Make sure your breath is smooth and flowing. If not, then rescue the twist so you can breathe better.

7. Hold for thirty seconds to one minute, then release by drawing the left knee back up to center and centering your head.

8. Release the legs out straight, and let the body settle.

9. When you are ready, repeat on the other side.

Adjusting and Twisting Using the Gym Ball

I find that, once again, the gym ball is a fabulous tool for dynamic forms of twisting and adjusting. Just be sure if you use the gym ball to make sure you are using your hands to keep yourself stable, and move slowly so you can keep yourself balanced when moving into any twisting or adjusting position.
The following pictures and descriptions are designed specifically for adjusting the lower and middle back. Remember, when moving into any twist, be sure to move on the exhale, not the inhale.

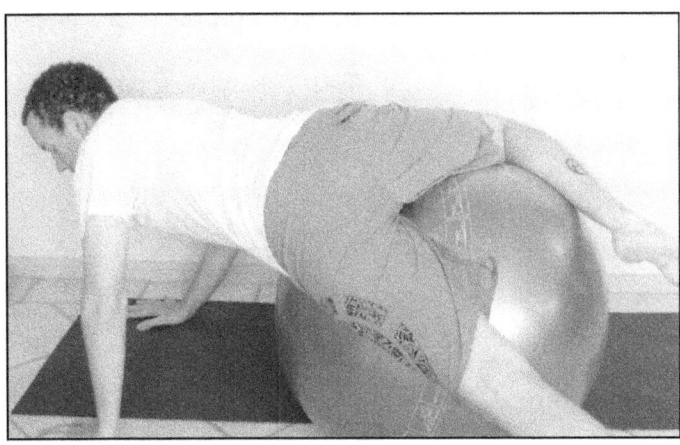

1. After you have spent some time lengthening your connective tissue to create space between the vertebrae, move the ball so it is down in the groin area.

2. Bend your knees slightly out to the side so as to stabilize your hips on top of the ball, and get your hands out wide on the floor so you can keep a steady balance as you move into the twist.

3. Begin to slowly roll the ball over to the left on a smooth and steady exhale breath. Be sure to use your upper-body strength and arms to keep you balanced.

4. You can make slight adjustments to the ball and hips to allow the twist to get all the areas of the lower back. You may get a pop or you may not; both are ok.

5. Generally, you don't stay in this position for any longer than ten seconds.

6. To release, just use your arms and the weight of the right leg to draw you back to the center position.

7. When you are ready, repeat this process on the other side.

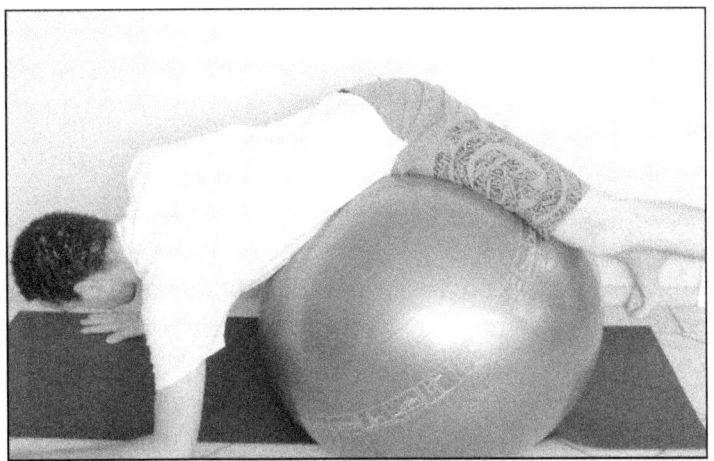

4. Lubricate and Nourish

Step four simply advises you to put good quality water into the body after any massage, yoga, movement, or treatment. This encourages fluids to flush through the newly "opened" area of the body. One of the aims of an adjustment or a release is to nourish the area with blood and nutrients so that the area can be properly healed and rejuvenated, because it is likely that that area has had little blood flow through it for some time. Therefore, always drink some water after an adjustment. It is better to drink room-temperature water or warm water than to drink ice-cold water, as ice-cold water is harder to digest and absorb into your system.

When working with any joints of the body, it is highly recommended that you supplement with fish oil, or omega-3 oils. These supplements help to lubricate the joints and reduce any pain associated with inflammation. Omega-3 oils also support a healthy nervous system, and can work to enhance brain function.

Magnesium is a natural muscle relaxant, and is worth taking if you are prone to tight muscles or the inability to relax your body. They can also help greatly with anxiety, stress, withdrawal symptoms, and insomnia. Be sure to try magnesium supplements before taking pharmaceuticals for muscle aches and pains or insomnia.

5. *Reorganize and retrain the muscles and tissues for more effective and efficient movement*

This step refers to a sustained and long-term solution to any muscular or skeletal problems, especially pain issues. The main cause of pain in the musculoskeletal system is having inefficient habitual movement patterns, which also contributes to incorrect or unbalanced posture. Poor movement patterns contribute to compression in the joints that leads to more serious musculoskeletal problems further down the track.

Do you get tired from walking only a short distance? Does you back hurt when you sit at the computer desk? Does your back hurt when you bend over to pick something up? Does your body hurt when you get up out of a chair? Does your neck hurt when you turn to look behind you when reversing the car? Do your shoulders or joints produce sharp pains when you lift weights at the gym? If so, these are all signs of poor movement behaviors and patterns.

Correcting (or at least altering) movement behavior starts with moving your body in new ways. This automatically begins creating new neural networks within the brain as it starts to reorganize itself according to the new information coming in. If we can show the nervous system easier and more efficient ways to move our bodies, it will learn to code this into the body's system. If we don't show the nervous system new ways to move, or stimulate it to reorganize, it will simply continue to produce the movement patterns that are already set up.

There are a few really good methods to retrain movement behavior. Yoga, the Feldenkrais method, and tai chi are, I believe, by far the best. While fast rapid movements tend to work the cardiovascular and muscular systems of the body, it's the slower, awareness-based, gentle movements that allow the nervous system time to reorganize itself. Therefore, slamming yourself at a gym on heavy weights will probably do little for correcting movement behavior, and in many cases can just reaffirm inefficient movement and technique. Focusing on slow, non-strenuous, and repetitive movements is the best way to help reorganize movement behavior.

Yoga is offered in a variety of styles and ways, and therefore not all yoga should be considered the same. Each teacher and style tends to emphasize different things, and some may be suitable and helpful, whereas some may not. Yin yoga is focused specifically on connective tissue lengthening, and is recommended. Personally, I have found that yoga is very helpful for adjusting and reorganizing the larger portions of the body— but it's the Feldenkrais method and tai chi which are the best at getting into the little nitty-gritty areas of the body.

The Feldenkrias method can be done in a class where a qualified practitioner instructs you. It's a very gentle form of movement class, where you tend to lie on the floor on blankets and do simple repetitive movements. You can also get a series of one-on-one treatments from a Feldenkrias practitioner who, again, uses simple and repetitive movements (it is very relaxing and not painful or stressful). Feldenkrais practitioners have been through an intensive four-year training course, and are highly skilled and considered to be health professionals. Check out www.feldenkrais.com for more info about this amazing modality.

If you get back pain on and off, then yoga would be a good place to start. I would also advise at least a few sessions or classes of the Feldenkrais method to iron out the details.

If you are in constant pain, then I would recommend you start off with gentler methods of retraining like the Feldenkrais method, yin yoga, or tai chi. I would also advise seeking assistance from a qualified osteopath or acupuncturist.

If you are rarely in pain, then yoga and other forms of exercise would be good to keep your body limber, flexible, and strong. Be sure to always fine-tune your alignment and technique to avoid hyper-mobile joints, and to avoid injury in the near future. It is still worth getting looked over by an osteopath every now and then to keep things in good working order.

"It is health that is real wealth and not pieces of gold and silver."

~ Mahatma Gandhi

Other Supportive Practices

Here are a few other practices and techniques that may help support your musculoskeletal system back to health.

1. Moxibustion and Cupping

Moxibustion, commonly known as "moxa," comes from Oriental medicine and involves the placement of a hot herb (mainly mugwart) near the body to add heat into the body tissues. Moxibustion is a powerful technique in the hands of skilled practitioner that can help reduce muscle spasm and stiffness in a matter of moments. Moxibustion is unique because, when it is burned, it has been found to give off infrared waves which are seen by the body as healthy and nurturing, therefore the body will tend to absorb these rays with joy. Most Chinese or Oriental medicine clinics have practitioners who can use these herbs in a treatment.

Cupping is a technique more well-known then moxibustion and is also a technique used in Chinese and Oriental medicine. It has a number of purposes, one of the main ones being that, instead of pushing down pressure onto tissue like massage does, it does the opposite by sucking up or drawing up tissue so that blood and fluid can move through the tissue much easier. When blood and fluids can move through tissue more easily, the body is able to heal the tissues much more effectively, therefore making cupping an effective technique in the hands of a skilled practitioner.

2. Avoid Stagnation and Sedentary Lifestyles

The body is designed to move, and it performs and functions at its best when we move it about on a daily basis. Tissues, blood, and fluids tend to become stagnant in parts of the body that are not moved, and this commonly leads to the tissues getting stuck together; in extreme cases, tissue can become locked into position. We want to avoid this sticking together of tissues as much as possible, and we can easily avoid that if we go for regular and gentle walks on most days.

3. Get a Spinal and Postural Evaluation from a Health Professional such as a Chiropractor or Osteopath

Chiropractors and Osteopaths are masters of postural evaluations and can see abnormalities in seconds. Some chiropractors also have an x-ray machine on-site and can take an x-ray of your spine that can then provide you with a more detailed analysis of your spinal and bone health. Getting insight and advice from these health professionals can provide a lot of insight and help motivate you into a lifestyle to support your musculoskeletal health.

4. Check Your Diet

Long periods of consuming unhealthy and unwholesome foods can lead to all sorts of complications which impair the health and healing capacity of your musculoskeletal system. In some cases, especially in women, without the support of a healthy diet and lifestyle, essential minerals and vitamins are leeched out of the bones leaving them to become brittle, weak, and prone to breaks and inflammation. A general principle is to avoid the overconsumption of acidic foods (sodas, cigarettes, alcohol, meats, oily foods, etc.), as they tend to stress our nervous system and impair body function. Instead, opt for a diet rich in alkaline-based foods (vegetables, fruits, fresh food, water, etc.), as this will reduce stress on the nervous system, support bodily function, and generally increase the health of all body tissues.

5. Only Buy and Use Furniture that Supports a Healthy Posture

A lot of furniture in the marketplace is poorly designed because many designers are only interested in the fashionable trends of the seasons and have little to no understanding of the biomechanics of the human musculoskeletal system. Using poorly designed furniture on a daily basis can cause unnecessary stress on the joints and muscles of the body as well as impair proper and efficient breathing. Be sure to sit in chairs that allow the knees to be slightly lower than the hips and to avoid chairs and couches that sink down, for they tend to round out the back and unbalance the spine. I always encourage sitting on a cushion on the floor as a natural way to open the hips, strengthen the core, and balance the spine. The sooner and younger you are when you get into these simple habits, the better it will be for your musculoskeletal health in the long run.

6. Consider Psychological Factors as a Contributing Influence in Musculoskeletal Pain

In cases of chronic pain, it has been found that the brain physiology changes to accommodate pain signals in the nervous system. So much so that the brain literally rewires itself over time to adjust so that the pain eventually becomes a type of neurological pattern. The consequences of this is that, even after traditional methods of addressing and removing the cause of pain have been dealt with, the pain still remains largely due to the new wiring in the brain and nervous system. Therefore, in some cases, physiological techniques and methods can be employed as a way to help manage the ongoing experience of pain and, at the same time, start working at rewiring the brain with the goal of dampening out the intensity of the pain signals with the potential to eliminate the pain signals completely. This is exemplified in the fact that what behaviours we repeat daily and where we place our attention consistently are what dictate the way our brains wire up. Therefore in the case of pain, after we have addressed the so-called cause, we then can change our points of attention and daily behaviours in a way that encourage the nervous system to change its wiring so that the pain signals are de-emphasized and weakened. This is a relatively new frontier in the field of medicine and psychology, and it's looking promising.

Another method or technique that tends to help a lot of people with musculoskeletal pain which doesn't have an obvious cause is to use E.F.T. (Emotional Freedom Technique). It works by the tapping of acupuncture points on the body, while acknowledging and focusing on the pain or issue. It is through the stimulation of these points and energetic pathways in the body that it triggers a shift out of a stressful, energetic state, which may be due to suppressed emotional factors, and moves our system into a more neutral and balanced state. This technique is really worth exploring and trying if nothing else has provided you with real, lasting relief. The technique takes no longer then five minutes at a time, is completely free, and has no negative side effects. For the best chance of results, it is advised to practice E.F.T. a number of times on each issue and, in some rare cases, to seek out a health practitioner who specializes in the technique, as they are trained to uncover deeper roots of an issue that we may not be able to see ourselves. To learn the technique, there are hundreds of YouTube videos available; or you can visit Gary Craig's website (www.emofree.com), who is one of the founders of this technique, to download an instructional manual or view some free videos.

*"Take Care of your body.
It is the only place you have to live."*

~ Jim Rohn

Conclusion

Musculoskeletal health doesn't have to be complicated or expensive. Just taking the time to learn how to relax the muscles in the body, stretch the connective tissue, and do a few simple stretches to adjust the body most days can often be enough to avoid the dreaded slipped disc and other conditions caused by tightness and compression.

Let's summarize the five-step process of self-adjusting:

1. Relax and release the musculature

Find ways to activate the trigger points located all around the back and shoulders. You can do this by using applied pressure, long deep breathing, and focused awareness. Muscle fibers respond quickly to trigger point release and quick stretches. If we fail to release muscles soon after tightness or spasm has occurred, the muscle can remain in this state for years and is harder to release and reset. Therefore, be sure to regularly release muscles as they become tight and contracted.

2. Soften and lengthen connective tissue

Connective tissue takes longer to respond than muscle fibers, therefore we need to hold deep stretches for at least three minutes with the body in a relaxed state in order to get to the deeper layers of connective tissue. Connective tissue surrounds the spine, and easily tightens and compresses due to ongoing stress and lack of movement. To rehabilitate any compression-related conditions (like a slipped disc), the connective tissue needs to be lengthened so more space can be created between the bones.

3. Twist to adjust (with or without a pop)

Once the muscles in the area are relaxed and the connective tissue has created some space between the bones, we can move into a twist position on an exhale breath to get an adjustment. This is often accompanied by a popping sound. Hold the twist for about thirty seconds with a smooth breath.

4. Lubricate and nourish

It is very important to keep the body hydrated, especially after any adjustment or stretching has taken place. Be sure to drink plenty of filtered water after any treatment, class, or adjustment. Add supplements like omega-3 fish oils for lubrication and nerve function, and magnesium for the relaxation and recovery of muscle fibers.

5. Reorganize the body for more efficient movement

To address reoccurring musculoskeletal health problems and any ongoing pain symptoms, it is highly recommended that you relearn and reorganize your movement patterns. The reoccurrence of musculoskeletal problems is likely due to inefficient and poor movement behavior that was learned and established at a very early age. You can relearn how to move more efficiently through the Feldenkrais method (most highly recommended) and other supporting practices like Tai Chi and yoga. Learning how to move more efficiently can not only reduce or eliminate pain symptoms, but it can also enhance athletic and mental performance.

All the techniques discussed in this book will give you enough to work with to address many musculoskeletal problems. However, if something arises that you are unable to treat effectively, be sure to go and see your trusted health practitioner. It is best to get on top of any health concerns or stresses as they arise because, generally speaking, anything that persists after two weeks is starting to become a chronic condition and needs to be treated as soon as possible.

In any case, for ongoing maintenance and preventative measures, I would recommend seeing your trusted health professional at least once every two months or so. This will enable you to nip any problems in the bud before they escalate into chronic conditions, and will save you a lot of time and money down the track. The best approach to healthcare is a preventative one, so congratulations on reading this book, as it shows that you are being proactive in managing your own health!

~ May All Beings Be Happy ~

Other Titles by Author:

Chakra Balancing Made Simple and Easy

Meditation Made Simple

How to Do Restorative Yoga

The Complete Book of Oriental Yoga

The Little Book of Yin

How to Learn Acupuncture

www.ingramcontent.com/pod-product-compliance
Lightning Source LLC
Chambersburg PA
CBHW051821170526
45167CB00005B/2106